Medical Ozone
A Hidden Source
of Disease Prevention
and Treatment

Jacob Swilling, Ph.D.
Consulting Research Scientist

Know Your Options™
www.knowyouroptionscenter.com

KYO Publishing

www.kyopublishing.com

Know Your Options Wellness Center

Suite M-3 John Wayne Water Garden Suites

3151 Airway Ave

Costa Mesa, CA 92626

(714) 708-3600

www.knowyouroptionscenter.com

ISBN-13:978-0692381434

ISBN-10:0692381430

Table of Contents

The Importance of Oxygen 1
Depletion of Oxygen 1
Depletion of Atmospheric Oxygen 1
Ozone in the Atmosphere 2
Ozone Neglected Due to the Focus on Antibiotics 2
Oxygen, Ozone and Cancer 2
Ozone and Cancer 3
Ozone and Water 3
Ozone as a Disinfectant 3
Ozone and AIDs 4
Ozone, Viruses and Bacteria 4
Breakthrough Information about Ozone, Bacteria, Fungi and Viruses 4
Biological Effects of Ozone 5
Conditions Effectively Treated by Ozone 6
Oxygen is Necessary for the Completion of These Bodily Functions 6
Benefits of Oxygen 6
Impact of Low Oxygen 7
Thirteen Major Effects of Ozone on the Body by Dr. Frank Shallenberger 8
Twenty-Three Protocols of Ozone Administration 12
Home use 13
Source of Ozone 13
Properties of Medical Ozone 13
Ozone Improves Oxygen Metabolism 14
The Electromagnetic Effect of Ozone 14
Ozone Induces Specific Enzymes 15
Management of Stroke 15
Ozone Activates Immune System 15
Route of Administration and Safety 16
Therapeutic Indications 16
What Does Ozone Do? 17
How Does Ozone Work? 18
Inactivates Bacteria, Viruses, Fungi, Yeast and Protozoa 18
Enhancement of Circulation 18

Stimulation of Oxygen Metabolism   18
Formation of Peroxides   19
Dissolution of Malignant Tumors   19
Activation of the Immune System   19
Ozone and the Immune System   20
The Immune System and the Emotions   20
SuggestedProtocols   21
A Review of Ozone Applications   23
Ear Insufflation   23
Vaginal Insufflation   24
Rectal Insufflaton   24
Body Suit   25
Ozone Sauna   26
Ozonated Olive Oil   27
Bagging   28
Major Autohemotherapy   29
Enhancing the Outcome of Ozone Therapy   30
The Use Of Chelation Therapy In Combination with Ozone   31
The Potential of Ozone in Your Clinic   32
References   37
About the Author   40

Medical Ozone

This information is written for medical doctors. Information is compiled from the scientific literature and is not intended for application without proper training and equipment approved by the author.

This information is protected by copyright and may not be copied or duplicated in part or whole without the written approval of the author.

The Importance of Oxygen

Of all the chemical elements, oxygen is the most vital to the human body. We would survive for only minutes without oxygen. Oxygen is the life-giving, life-sustaining element. Approximately 90% of the body's energy is created by oxygen. Nearly all of the body's activities, from brain function to elimination, are regulated by oxygen. The ability to think, feel and act is derived from the basic energy supplied by oxygen.

The only way to truly optimize health is to ensure complete cellular oxygenation. Every one of the body's trillions of cells demands oxygen for proper function.

Depletion of Oxygen

Depletion of Atmospheric Oxygen

The oxygen-energy cycle has become critically important today, more than at any time in human history, because of the progressive and unnatural decrease in atmospheric oxygen.

There are many causes for this decrease in atmospheric oxygen such as deforestation, auto and industrial pollution, devitalized soil, volcanic eruptions and so on. It has been estimated that the air breathed by our distant ancestors contained approximately 45-50 % oxygen. Two hundred years ago, the air was composed of 38% oxygen and 10% carbon dioxide. The level measured by Swiss scientists in 1945-1946 was 22%. They have been carefully monitoring this level ever since. The most recent measurement was 19% with more than 25% carbon dioxide. In our major cities the oxygen level may be lower than 10%!

Ozone in the Atmosphere

Ozone is as essential to our lives as the air we breathe. Ozone purifies the lower atmosphere by combining with dangerous hydrocarbons, reducing them to harmless carbon dioxide and water.

Ozone shields us from deadly radiation in the upper atmosphere by forming the much-talked-about "ozone layer." The ancient Hebrews had an intuitive sense of the importance of ozone, referring to it as "the breath of God."

Ozone Neglected Due to the Focus on Antibiotics

The enormous expenditures made by giant pharmaceutical manufacturers on the development of antibiotics and other drugs has ensured that natural ozone, a more successful protocol, has been relegated to practices conducted in just a few countries, such as Germany and Russia.

However, recent reports estimate that more than 7,000 physicians in Europe, Canada, Israel, Australia, New Zealand, China, Korea, Cuba and the Philippines are using ozone.

Research by European doctors over several decades has proven conclusively that hyper-oxygenation of the blood through various modalities can restore even advanced states of illness and disease to vibrant health as well as slow or even reverse the aging process.

Proper oxidation makes the difference between health and a disease state.Insufficient oxygen means insufficient biological energy that can result in anything from mild fatigue to life-threatening illness.

Oxygen, Ozone and Cancer

Dr. Otto Warburg, twice a Nobel Laureate, was awarded

the Nobel Prize in 1931 for discovering the cause of cancer. He claimed that, "for cancer there is one prime cause ... the replacement of oxygen respiration in normal cells by the fermentation of sugar." In other words, the growth of cancer cells is initiated by a relative lack of oxygen. Furthermore, cancer cells cannot live in an oxygen-rich environment.

This research was continued by Dr. Harry Goldblatt, who published his findings in 1953. His research concluded that a lack of oxygen plays a major role in causing cells to become cancerous.

In another study, cancer cell growth inhibition was 90% when exposed to only .8 ppm (parts per million) of ozone.

Ozone and Cancer

Ozone is the most effective source capable of delivering oxygen through the blood to restore oxygen to anaerobic cells. Otto Warburg won the Nobel prize in 1948 for demonstrating that the primary cause of cancer is the replacement of oxygen in the respiratory chemistry of normal cells by the fermentation of sugar. The growth of cancer cells is a fermentation process which can be initiated only in the relative absence of oxygen.

Other important research demonstrates that cancer growths contract and disappear when the oxygen saturation is sufficiently increased in the fluids surrounding them.

Ozone and Water

Ozone has been employed as a safe and effective water purifier for more than a century. It rapidly destroys viruses, bacteria and fungi as well as spores, moulds, cysts and yeast. It oxidizes chemicals and pollutants including fluorine, chlorine, and THMs, yielding crystal pure, sterile water.

Ozone as a Disinfectant

Ozone is the second most powerful disinfectant known. Ozone kills bacterial and viral pathogens such as E. Coli more than 3,125 times faster than chlorine, and without the carcinogenic side effects. There are currently several thousand water treatment plants worldwide using ozone to purify their water resources.

Ozone and AIDS

Ozone therapy has been in use by hundreds of West German doctors who claim in numerous clinical studies that they are able to inactivate AIDS and other viruses, as well as cancer through ozone therapy.

Ozone, Viruses and Bacteria

Many other studies have reported evidence that viruses and bacteria cannot survive the impact of oxygen.

Healthy cells need oxygen. Most infections occur because of the invasion of anaerobes that do not thrive in an oxygen environment.

In other research studies, evidence suggests that when calves and pigs were kept in sheds designed to promote good air circulation and maintain the full complement of oxygen, a virus could hardly travel a meter. However, when the oxygen level was lowered by only a few percent, a virus could circulate freely.

Other research studies have demonstrated that homes and offices closed up in winter to retain heat and in summer to keep cool (especially those with central heating/air conditioning) became "sick" buildings. They became traps for viruses because of stale oxygen-reduced air and those that live or work in them had higher rates of illness.

Breakthrough Information about Ozone, Bacteria, Fungi and Viruses

Ozone therapy has been used in this century to kill bacteria, fungi and viruses in the body for more than 75 years. In one study, the poliovirus was exposed to .21 mg/ liter of ozone. After only 30 seconds, 99% of the viruses were inactivated.

Viruses are not cells. They are either RNA or DNA genetic material, not both. Since they have only half of the required genetic material, they cannot reproduce on their own.

As a result of poor nutrition and/or environmental stress, normal cells become diseased. These cells are an opportunity for a virus to penetrate them. The viruses attach themselves to the inner RNA or DNA of these "host" cells and then use the genetic material inside the cell to replicate themselves.

As these viruses multiply, their metabolic waste begins to overwhelm the body's ability to eliminate it, resulting in illness.

Outside of their host cell viruses are inert. They "hide out" inside the cell and must be uncovered in order to be destroyed.

This is where the amazing property of ozone is so effective because it can invade diseased cells, and uncover and destroy viruses. Ozone, because it possesses that third atom of oxygen, is "electrophilic." It is a radical that seeks to balance itself electrically with other material that has a corresponding unbalanced charge. Diseased cells, viruses, harmful bacteria and other pathogens carry such a charge, and so attract ozone and its by-products.

Biological Effects of Ozone

Regular use of ozone therapy strengthens the immune system by enhancing circulation, providing an oxygen-rich environment for cellular rejuvenation, cleansing the blood of impurities, clearing plaque from the arteries, optimizing the acid/alkaline balance of the body, improving nutrient assimilation and by removing putrefactive deposits from the intestines and colon.

These and many other beneficial results of ozone therapy make ozone ideal for rejuvenation and life extension and perhaps the most effective means for reversing the "aging process."

Conditions Effectively Treated by Ozone

What follows is a brief list of conditions that have been effectively treated with ozone therapy.

Candida and Epstein-Barr, AIDS, hepatitis, cancer, Multiple Sclerosis (M.S.), Alzheimer's, heart and arterial Diseases, acne, allergies, anal fissures, arterial circulatory disturbances, arteriosclerosis, arthritis, arthrosis, athlete's foot, bed sores, bronchial asthma, burns, cerebral sclerosis, cirrhosis of the liver, circulatory disturbances (venous and arterial), irritable colon, constipation, cystitis, dental conditions, fistulae, fungus infections, gangrene, genital infections, geriatrics, hemorrhage,herpes genital, herpes labialis, herpes zoster (shingles), hypercholesterolemia, immuno-stimulation, joint complaints, oral disease, stomatitis, mycosis, oncological support treatment, orthopedics, osteomyelitis, Parkinson's Disease, polyarthritis, radiation scars, Raynoud's Disease, RES insufficiency, skin infections, thrombophlebitis, ulcus cruris, varicosis, wound healing.

This is by no means an exhaustive list of the conditions for which ozone therapy has been successfully applied.

Oxygen is Necessary for the Completion of These Bodily Functions

- Food digestion
- Nutritional assimilation
- Waste removal
- Supply of energy to the muscles
- The manufacture and growth of muscles
- Cell growth and repair

Benefits of Oxygen

- Elimination of Chronic Fatigue

- Enhances circulation
- Activates the immune system
- Normalization of cell respiration
- Restoration of normal metabolism
- Elimination of Fibromyalgia
- Prevents the absorption of toxins into the body
- Enhances the effectiveness of ongoing treatments
- Eliminates bacteria, viruses, and fungus
- Leaves you relaxed and feeling good
- Removes toxins from the surface of the skin as well as the pores

Impact of Low Oxygen

The body is designed to function optimally at 100% oxygen saturation. Oxygen levels in those considered healthy, range from 96% to 98%. The evidence is that those suffering from chronic illness have oxygen levels as low as 85%. At these levels, oxygen in the body is so low as to cause the development of fermentation leading to the development of yeast, fungus, bacteria, viruses and parasites.

This cumulative effect results in depletion of available nutrients needed by the body as a living organism. Further, the excretion of their wastes drains the immune system and accelerates illness and disease of the body.

Deprivation of oxygen to the body, occurs through polluted air, sedentary lifestyle, poor posture and shallow breathing. Poor nutrition or a junk food diet requires a greater amount of oxygenation to eliminate waste products and encourages anaerobic microbes to proliferate. Overgrowth of harmful microbes will lead to breakdown of enzymatic reactions, overload of metabolic wastes and ultimately cell death.

Under similar anaerobic conditions, cells tend to mutate to

more primitive life forms, turning from aerobic to anaerobic respiration for energy synthesis.

Thirteen Major Effects of Ozone on the Body by Dr. Frank Shallenberger

Ozone stimulates the production of white blood cells. These cells protect the body from viruses, bacteria, fungi and cancer. Deprived of oxygen, these cells malfunction. They fail to eliminate invaders and even turn against normal, healthy cells (causing reactions like allergies). Ozone significantly raises oxygen levels in the blood for long periods after ozone administration; as a result, allergies have a tendency to become desensitized.

Interferon levels are significantly increased. Interferons are globular proteins. Interferons orchestrate every aspect of the immune system. Some interferons are produced by cells infected by viruses. These interferons warn adjacent, healthy cells of the likelihood of infection; in turn, they are rendered non permissive host cells. In other words, they inhibit viral replication. Other interferons are produced in the muscles, connective tissue and by white blood cells. Levels of gamma interferon can be elevated 400-900% by ozone. This interferon is involved in the control of phagocytic cells that engulf and kill pathogens and abnormal cells.

Interferons are FDA-approved for the treatment of chronic Hepatitis Band C, genital warts (caused by Papillomavirus), hairy cell leukemia, Kaposi's sarcoma, Relapsing-Remitting Multiple Sclerosis (RRMS) and Chronic Granulomatous Disease (CGD). Interferons are currently in clinical trials for throat warts (caused by Papillomavirus), HIV infection, Chronic Myelogenous Leukemia, Non-Hodgkin's Lymphoma (NHL), colon tumors, kidney tumors, bladder cancer, malignant melanoma, basal cell carcinoma (BCC) and Leishmaniasis. While levels induced by ozone remain safe, interferon levels that are FDA-approved (and in clinical trials) are extremely toxic.

Ozone stimulates the production of tumor necrosis factor (TNF). TNF is one of a number of proteins produced to destroy tumors growing in the body. The greater the tumor mass, the more tumor necrosis factor is produced. When a tumor has turned metastatic, cancer cells are breaking off and being carried away by the blood and lymph. This allows the tumor to take up residence elsewhere in the body; or in other words, divide its forces.

These lone cancer cells have little chance of growing due to the TNF produced to inhibit the original tumor. However, when a tumor is removed surgically, TNF levels drop dramatically afterward due to the diminished threat. Sometimes new tumors emerge from seemingly healthy tissue after the TNF drops if conditions in the body are conducive.

Ozone stimulates the secretion of IL-2. Interluekin-2 is one of the cornerstones of the immune system. It is secreted by T-helpers. In a process known as auto-stimulation, the IL-2 then binds to a receptor on the T-helper and causes it to produce more IL-2. Its main duty is to induce lymphocytes to differentiate and proliferate, yielding more T-helpers, T-suppressors, cytotoxic T's, T-delayed's and T-memory cells.

Ozone is able to kill most bacteria at low concentration because the metabolism of most bacteria is on average one-seventeenth as efficient as our body's metabolism. Very few types of bacteria can live in an environment composed of more than two percent ozone.

When the immune system is compromised there is not enough capacity to make antioxidant enzymes such as catalase that can counter the negative effects of harmful bacteria.

Ozone is effective against all types of fungi. This includes systemic Candida albicans, athlete's foot, molds, mildews, yeasts and even mushrooms.

Ozone fights viruses in a variety of ways. As discussed above, ozone also goes after the viral particles directly. The part of the virus most sensitive to oxidation is the reproductive structure.

When ozone enters the cell it destroys the capacity of the virus to reproduce. With this structure inactivated, the virus is essentially "dead." The virus has a natural weakness to ozone. With the metabolic burden of the virus, the body's cells can no longer produce enzymes necessary to deal with the infection and repair the cell. With ozone treatment, the cells are relieved of the burden of infection and can devote attention to repair and healing of the body.

Ozone is antineoplastic, it inhibits the growth of new cancer tissue because rapidly dividing cells shift their priorities away from reproducing to protecting themselves from the ozone. Cancer cells are then inhibited by ozone.

Ozone oxidizes arterial plaque. It breaks down the plaque involved in both arteriosclerosis and atherosclerosis. This means ozone has a tendency to clear blockages of large and even smaller vessels. This allows for better tissue oxygenation in deficient organs.

Ozone increases the flexibility and elasticity of red blood cells. When one views a red blood cell under a microscope, it looks like a disc. In the capillaries, where they pick-up and release oxygen, these discs stretch out into the shape of an oval or umbrella. This aids their passage through the tiny vessels and allows oxygen levels to stay elevated for days, even weeks after treatment with ozone.

Ozone accelerates the citric acid cycle. Also known as the Kreb's cycle or tricarboxylic acid cycle (TCA) cycle, this is a very important step in the glycolysis of carbohydrate for energy. This takes place in the mitochondria of the cell. Most of the energy stored in glucose (sugar) is converted in this pathway.

Ozone makes the antioxidant enzyme system more efficient and degrades petrochemicals. These chemicals have a potential to place a great burden on the immune system, and even causing allergies that are detrimental to long-term health.

Note: Considered one of the leading authorities on medical ozone, Dr. Shallenberger has done important work to support the hypothesis that ozone can have long-term positive effects on AIDS. He has also conducted workshops on the proper application of medical ozone at an international ozone symposium in Texas. He successfully treats patients' with medical ozone via major autohemotherapy.

Twenty-Three Protocols of Ozone Administration

There are twenty-three methods of administering medical ozone in the clinic. They are:

1. Intravenous injection
2. Intra arterial injection
3. Direct injection into a tumor
4. Autohemotherapy
5. Intracutaneous blistering
6. Intramuscularly
7. Subcutaneous
8. Uterine insufflation
9. Bladder insufflation
10. Subatmospheric
11. Bagging
12. Dental use of ozonated water
13. Rectal insufflation
14. Vaginal insufflation
15. Drinking water
16. In the ear
17. Ozonated water enema
18. Breathing through olive oil
19. Deep lymphatic massage with ozonated olive oil
20. Ozonated bath with Epsom Salts and sea salt
21. Body suit
22. Steam cabinet
23. External limb bagging

Home Use

There is evidence of an increasing number of patients using ozone in the home. Ozone equipment and know-how supplied by clinics is being used at home in response to demand from patients for the following reasons:

Ozonated water to wash vegetables

Ozonated water as disinfectant

Ozonated water used for enemas

Ozonated steam bath

Ozonated olive oil for topical use

Ozonated bath water

In addition in special circumstance when patients need daily treatment for an extended period for pathological conditions, the use of ozone bagging for the treatment of gangrene limbs as well as insufflations for the ear, rectal and vaginal applications. These home treatments are carefully monitored requiring regular visits for evaluation.

Source of Ozone

The same ozone in the atmospheric layer that is responsible for shielding from ultra-violet light from the sun and oxidizing the pollutants in the air can be produced from medical oxygen via electrical discharge.

Such ozone is administered as an ozone/oxygen gas mixture. According to the dosage and concentration range, medical ozone is a potent healing agent that exerts specific healing properties in a well-defined range of efficacy.

Properties of Medical Ozone

At the highest range of concentration (3.5 to 5%, ozone in a one/oxygen mixture) ozone exhibits a strong germicidal effect by oxidative destruction. The oxidative power of ozone has proven to be effective in destroying lipid-enveloped viruses such as Epstein-Barr, herpes, cytomegalovirus and viruses that cause hepatitis. One study reports that ozone treatment was 97-to-100% effective in destroying HIV in vitro. (Journal of American Society of Haematology, October 1, 1992).

At concentrations below approximately 3.5%, the three main restorative properties of ozone can be observed by its oxidative influence on the oxygen metabolism, the generation of specific enzymes and the activation of immuno-competent cells. It is these systematic influences of ozone that cause it to be such a potent therapeutic procedure, as most of the diseases affecting humans today can be traced to diminished levels of oxygen and a compromised immune system.

Ozone Improves Oxygen Metabolism

Ozone improves the delivery of oxygen to hypoxic tissues (hypoxic reduction of oxygen to tissue below physiological levels despite adequate perfusion of the tissue by blood), as well as reactivating the oxygen metabolism of cells. The mechanisms of these systemic actions involves both direct and indirect processes.

The Electromagnetic Effect of Ozone

Ozone directly changes the electric charges of the erythrocyte membrane increasing the flexibility and mobility of the erythrocytes, thus enhancing the flow properties of the blood and the transport of oxygen to cells and tissues. This is especially applicable in arterial occlusion disease whereby stacked erythrocyte formation typically looks like a "pile of coins." The indirect mechanism consists of ozonolysis, i.e., the ionizing reaction of ozone with the unsaturated fatty acids in the cellular membrane producing peroxides.

Ozone behaves as an ion, not a free radical under normal physiological blood pH and therefore no radical chain reaction occurs to cause oxidative damages. The reaction activates the enzyme 2, 3Diphosphoglycerate (2, 3-DPG) in hemoglobin to release oxygen. This is of particular importance in diabetics in which 2, 3-DPG is depressed.

Ozone Induces Specific Enzymes

These short-lived peroxides at the membrane enter into the cell and are removed by the enzyme glutathione peroxidase. Therefore, it is recommended to supplement with vitamin E, N-acetylcysteine (NAC) and selenium during ozone. In addition, the enhancement of the glycolysis enzymatic pathway results in an increase in adenosine triphosphate production (ATP, energy currency of the cell).

Management of Stroke

In a forthcoming book, Dr. Swilling will describe the life-saving impact of ATP on stroke and burns.

The elevation of adenosine triphosphate synthesis will decrease perifocal edema formed at an injured site, minimizing tissue necrosis and subsequent scarring. With injury, it is crucial that ozone is administered within the first 24-to-48 hours. In Germany, many ambulances are equipped with ozone and it is administered intravenously in patients who have just suffered a stroke.

Ozone Activates Immune System

It is well documented that ozone can activate monocytes and lymphocytes and induce the production of a variety of cytokines such as interleukin, interferon, necrosis-necrosis factor. (The Journal of International Medical Research 1994). Its ability to elicit endogenous production of cytokines and its lack of toxicity make ozone an indispensable therapeutic modality because today's most devastating diseases are characterized by immuno-depression, with such chronic diseases as cancer and AIDS. Of course, restoration of the immune system depends on a total approach of detoxification, lifestyle change, therapeutic nutrition and supportive therapies.

Route of Administration and Safety

There are several methods used to administer ozone, depending upon the condition being treated. Autohemotherapy, which involves treatment ex vivo of blood with ozone and prompt reinfusion, is the most popular procedure among German physicians. Other methods include direct infusion of a gaseous ozone/oxygen mixture either intravenously or intra-arterially (particularly in critical limb ischemia)

It has been proven that even direct delivery of ozone into the blood vessels has very low risk factors. No air which contains nitrogen ever enters the body so an air embolus cannot occur. Colorectal insufflation of ozone/oxygen much like an enema, has been used to treat colitis, fistula and colon cancer.

Ozone is also excellent for topical treatment of infected wounds, gangrene, ulcers and burns, especially those that are difficult to heal.

Therapeutic Indications

The modern development of ozone application in medicine began in the 1950s in Europe and gradually spread to Australia, Israel, Cuba, Brazil and Columbia. As far back as World War I, ozone was used medically to treat wounds and other infections. Now, over 7000 physicians world- wide routinely use ozone in their practice of medicine.

The author has monitored several hundred ozone-treated cancer patients all of whom reported beneficial changes and demonstrated improved blood and immune response. When it is incorporated into an integrated health care treatment approach,there is virtually no known side effect of ozone treatment if it is applied properly. However, since ozone therapy is dose-dependent, it should be administered only with the supervision of experienced medical staff.

Other than cancer, specific therapeutic applications of ozone include treatment of vascular disease, such as stroke, obstructive arteriopathy, venous insufficiency, cancer, acute and chronic viral diseases, ulcers, infected wounds, gangrene, burns, inflammatory bowel disease such as Crohn's disease, ulcerative colitis and spinal disc problems.

It is also used in dentistry as a disinfectant and in pediatrics for the treatment of viral and bacterial infections of the intestines. In geriatrics, its principal indication is in circulatory disorders. In particular, the increase of oxygen supply to the brain is of great benefit.

Ozone, with all its miraculous properties and accompanied by its lack of toxicity, is undoubtedly an important therapy in medicine. It is unusual in its dual capacity to defend the body via its stimulation of the immune system and at the same time improve oxygenation and metabolism.

What Does Ozone Do?

- Inactivates viruses, bacteria, yeast, fungus and protozoa
- Stimulates the immune system
- Cleans arteries and veins, improves circulation
- Purifies the blood and lymph
- Normalizes hormone and enzyme production
- Reduces inflammation
- Reduces pain
- Calms the nerves
- Stops bleeding
- Prevents shock
- Prevents stroke damage
- Reduces cardiac arrhythmia
- Improves brain function and memory
- Oxidizes toxins, allowing their excretion
- Chelates heavy metals; it works well in conjunction with EDTA

- Prevents and reverses degenerative diseases
- Prevents and treats communicable diseases
- Prevents and eliminates autoimmune diseases

Ozone, with all its miraculous properties and accompanied by its lack of toxicity, is undoubtedly an important therapy in medicine. It is an unusual double-edged sword. It defends the body via its stimulation of the immune system and at the same time it improves oxygenation and metabolism.

How Does Ozone Work?

Inactivates bacteria, viruses, fungi, yeast and protozoa

Ozone disrupts the integrity of the bacterial cell envelope through oxidation of the phospholipids and lipoproteins. In fungi, ozone inhibits cell growth at certain stages. With viruses, the ozone damages the viral capsid and disrupts the reproductive cycle by disrupting the virus-to-cell contact with peroxidation. The weak enzyme coatings on cells which make them vulnerable to invasion by viruses make them susceptible to oxidation and elimination from the body, and then replaces them with healthy cells.

Enhancement of circulation

In circulatory disease, a clumping of red cells hinders movement through the small capillaries and decreases oxygen absorption due to reduced surface area. Ozone reduces or eliminates clumping and red cell flexibility is restored, along with oxygen carrying ability. Oxygenation of the tissues increases as the arterial pressure increases and viscosity decreases. Ozone also oxidizes the plaque in arteries, allowing the removal of the breakdown these products, and unclogging the blood vessels.

Stimulation of oxygen metabolism

Ozone causes an increase in the red blood cell glycolysis rate. This leads to the stimulation of 2,3-diphosphoglycerate

(2,3-DPG) which leads to an increase in the amount of oxygen released into the tissues. There is a stimulation of the production of the enzymes which act as free radical scavengers and cell wall protectors, including glutathione peroxidase, catalase, and superoxide dismutase.

Ozone activates the Krebs Cycle by enhancing oxidative carboxilation of pyruvate, stimulating production of ATP. Ozone also causes a reduction in NADH and helps to oxidize cytochrome c prostacycline, a vasodilator, that is also induced by ozone.

Formation of peroxides

Ozone reacts with the unsaturated fatty acids of the lipid layer in cellular membranes, forming hydro peroxides. There is a synergistic effect with cellular-formed H202. Lipid peroxidation products include alkoxyl and peroxyl radicals, singlet oxygen, ozonides, carbonyls, alkanes and alkenes.

Dissolution of malignant tumors

Ozone inhibits tumor metabolism. In addition, ozone oxidizes the outer lipid layer of malignant cells and destroys them through cell lysis. Phagocytes produce H202 and hydroxyl to kill bacteria and viruses. The generation of hydroxyl of L-arginine to citrulline, nitrite and nitrates by phagocytes, acts upon the tumors.

Activation of the immune system

Ozone administered at a concentration of about 50 ug/cc causes the greatest increase in the production of interferon. Higher or lower concentrations have a correspondingly lower effect. Interleukin tumor necrosis factor (TNF) is released in the greatest quantities between 30 and 50 ug/cc. The production of interleukin-2 launches an entire cascade of subsequent immunological reactions.

Ozone and the Immune System

Ozone is not a drug and it is not a magic bullet. It is a therapeutic procedure of great power which can aid the body in regaining health. However, in the end, it is the immune system that has to do the work of healing the body. Therefore, the immune system must be viable.

The immune system and the emotions

The immune system is controlled by the midbrain, the limbic system, through the thymus. The limbic system also controls the emotions. If the emotions are disrupted, the immune system is suppressed or shut down.

Research by Dr. Glen Rein at HeartMath has shown that the thymus, the "general of the army" of the immune system, is regulated by sympathetic resonance with the heartbeat. By measuring the regularity of the heartbeat with an electrocardiogram, Dr. Rein was able to show that an irregular heartbeat, as caused by emotional upset, produced erratic thymus function, which suppressed the immune system. Dr. Rein also found that it was possible to train people to control their heartbeat and raise their level of immune function.

Since ozone has a well known calming and analgesic effect, due to restoring heartbeat regularity, perhaps ozone therapy has a role to play in enhancing the immune system, along with interleukin-2 stimulation. Ozone is already used as a treatment for heart arrhythmia.

Therefore prolonged used of ozone would enhance the immune system by contributing to a calm, even heartbeat, produced by a well-oxygenated heart pumping clean bright red blood through plaque-free arteries.

Suggested protocols:

Direct tumor injection - such as a breast tumor.

1-10 injections required; needle aspiration, liquefaction increases as the concentration of ozone increases, sometimes the installation of a continuous drain is required, sometimes just a poultice.

Vagina, uterus

Catheter adiministration with humidfication; endometritis requires insertion of catheter into cervical os.

Ear insufflation

For infections; five minutes per ear with humidification.

Direct intravenous injection

Ozone is injected into the portal (rectal) vein for cancer (especially liver cancer) and hepatitis; it is suggested to administer an EDTA-type of chelation as well.

Autohemotherapy

Use a syringe or bottle.

Nasal inhalation

20 ug/ml of ozone through 2″ olive oil for 15 minutes twice daily.

Rectal insufflation

Use about 500ml in one minute spurts to induce retroperistalsis to prevent gas pains. Slow continuous administration is also satisfactory, humidification is required.

Hyperbaric

10ug/cc/ozone at pressure - 30 - 35 psi.

The potency of any medicine is greatly increased when taken in conjunction with ozone therapy, e.g. aspirin 100 times;

chemotherapy 10 times.

Hydrogen peroxide injection

Mixed results, it is suggested to keep amounts and concentrations low - 0.375%.

Ozonated steam cabinet

Especially effective method of treating the lymph system.

External limb bagging

A Review of Ozone Applications

Ear Insufflation

Many individuals have found it beneficial to irrigate the ear with the ozone/oxygen mixture from a medical ozone generator. As with every use of ozone for medical purposes, the individual must ensure: the purity of the oxygen supply, and that all parts of the ozone generator that are in contact with the gas stream are ozone resistant (e.g, Kynar, Teflon, glass, silicon) and they must know the ozone concentration of the ozone generator. This is extremely important - too little ozone and there will be no effect; too much ozone and there can be irritation in the ear canal.

The patient may first apply a small amount of water to the ear canal to assist in the absorption of the ozone. The ozone must be humidified by bubbling the gas through the water.

The usual concentration used for this protocol is 15ug/ml - 30 ug/ml. The flow rate used is usually 1/4 liter per minute or perhaps 1/8 LPM (liters per minute).

The output tube of the ozone generator is held up to the entrance of the ear. At no time should the tube come into proximity with the eyes, nose or mouth. Doing so may cause discomfort. At no time should the output tube be placed inside the ear, or sealed into the entrance way of the ear.

The ozone should be allowed to flow into the ear and out the ear. Each ear is usually treated for 2-5 minutes per treatment.

Treatment schedule depends on the disease of the patient, and the effect the ozone therapy is having on each individual patient. This therapy should not be performed more than once per day, and in most cases is performed 2-3 times per week.

The therapist should individually modify the treatment protocol depending on patient reaction~ If any discomfort, redness, or chapping occurs, it is suggested that the patient increase the length of time between treatments, and decrease the ozone concentration coming from the ozone generator.

Many physicians have indicated that the ozone enters the lymphatic and blood system using this treatment protocol. Many patients have reported a wide variety of results including relief from allergies and colds, clearing of sore throats and swollen glands.

Vaginal insufflation

A vaginal cannula is used to introduce ozone gas into the patient. Unlike rectal insufflation, there is no danger of pressure buildup. The ozone concentration used is usually 25-30 ug/ml, and the flow rate is usually 1/4 LPM (liters per minute) or 1/8 LPM. Treatment time is usually 5-15 minutes. The patient may lower the ozone concentration and the duration of the treatment if any discomfort occurs. This treatment should not be performed more than once per day, and is usually only performed 2-3 times per week.

Many women have reported relief from yeast infections and various sexually transmitted diseases including herpes. Many women also use this method as an alternative to rectal insufflation, because it is theorized that the ozone not only affects the pelvic region, but also enters into general circulation, causing a body wide effect.

Women must not use this method close to or during the time of menstruation as ozone at these concentrations increases blood flow.

Rectal insufflation

Rectal insufflation is "95% as effective as major autohemotherapy," per Dr. Renate Viebahn. This method is used by many physicians in their clinics and by those at home as well.

The ozone gas (usually at a concentration between 20 ug/ml — 35 ug/ml, and a flow rate of 1/8 liter per minute) is infused rectally using a urethral catheter. The procedure is usually performed following a bowel movement or a colonic treatment in order to ensure the colon is relatively free of fecal matter. The ozone enters the lower intestine, is held for at least thirty minutes, and over this period it is absorbed into the system.

This type of treatment is performed at initially high concentration and gradually lowered as treatments continue for such problems as colitis, bacterial infections, or bleeding. The treatment is performed using the above guidelines, but with a lower in concentration, if the desired effects are the immune modulation and other 'system wide' effects typically desired of Ozone Therapy.

Infusing gas rectally is much like blowing up a balloon. For safety and comfort reasons the physician and patient must always ensure that only the desired volume of ozone gas is infused. A typical starting point for many users is 125 cc of gas (which can be obtained if the flow rate is 1/8 liter per minute as above, and the treatment is performed for one minute).

The ozone gas is infused through the catheter which is inserted into the rectum approximately 4 to 6 inches. Using the example above, the flow is then stopped within one minute, the catheter withdrawn, and the patient then holds this gas for a period of at least thirty minutes.

Why thirty minutes? Dr. Michael Carpendale has shown through studies that the ozone gas is absorbed over a period of thirty-to-forty minutes as it is held in the body. If the ozone escapes before this time, the full benefit of the treatment will not been obtained. The gas must be slowly absorbed into the body for the system wide effects of ozone therapy to be obtained. Most users have mentioned that little or no discomfort is caused by this method, and most find they have no gas release at the end of the thirty minute period.

Body suit

One of the easiest and most pleasurable of methods of using ozone, the body suit is both effective and relaxing. Ozone is absorbed through the skin, cleansing the lymphatic system, and reportedly inducing body-wide effects of ozone generally seen with other treatment protocols.

The patient first opens the pores of the skin by taking a warm/ hot shower after which they immediately enter the body suit.

The body suit must be sealed at the ankles and wrists to reduce leaking. Usually a towel is wrapped around the neck to increase comfort and to reduce leaking around the neck. If necessary, a fan may be used to gently blow any leaking ozone away from the individual.

The ozone generator is set to produce a concentration of 25-35 ug/ml at a flow rate of 1/4 LPM. The ozone must first be humidified (run through water) before it is introduced into the body suit.

The patient remains in the body suit for fifteen-forty minutes (One usually starts with a fifteen minute treatment. The treatment time remains the same amount of time or is gradually increased depending on the desire and comfort of the individual during and after treatments). Treatment is usually individualized depending on the individual effects of the treatments and the desired effect, be it in treatment of a disease, or for general health. Individuals should be encouraged to use their own bodies and common sense to guide the treatment times and concentrations should be increased or lowered. This treatment is usually performed 2-3 times per week, and never more than once a day.

Ozone sauna

The benefits of a sauna on the immune system and disease processes have been well documented. In addition to being relaxing and soothing, a sauna and the accompanying induced hyperthermia on the body, mimics the beneficial effects of fever without the discomfort. At 104 degrees F., for example, the growth rate of the polio virus is reduced up to 250 times, at 106 degrees pneumococcus, a bacterium responsible for pneumonia, dies.

Although the effects of this artificial method of increasing body temperature are not as comprehensive as a natural fever there are definite system-wide effects. There is evidence that this artificial method works as an immune system stimulant to increase the number of white blood cells in the body.

In a 1959-review of studies on the effects of heat treatment, Mayo Clinic researcher Dr. Watkin and colleagues cite findings indicating that the number of white blood cells in the blood increased by an average of 58% during artificially-induced fever. Researchers also have found increases in the activity of the white blood cells during induced fever.

Apart from the immune system-stimulating effects of sweat therapy, many have thought it to be one of the most effective and painless detoxifying treatments available. Sweat contains almost the same elements as urine, and for this reason, the skin is sometimes called the third kidney. It is estimated that as much as 30% of bodily wastes are eliminated by way of perspiration, and during a steam sauna, the body perspires profusely.

By adding ozone into this environment, the ozone is easily absorbed into the skin and lymphatic system because of the open pores. This provides an excellent detoxifying effect and it is also reported that the effects are those that are desired in the medical use of ozone.

It is very important to point out that the sauna used for this treatment is of the type where the individual's head protrudes from the top of the sauna, and the individual is therefore not breathing the ozone/steam mixture. Concentrations used for this type of treatment are usually approximately 40ug/ml and the ozone is introduced into the sauna at a rate of 1/4LPM. One should remain in the sauna for fifteen-thirty minutes, but never longer. Taking a steam sauna has many beneficial effects, but as in most cases, more is not necessarily better — thirty minutes is maximum whether ozone is used or not.

Ozonated olive oil

Ozonated Olive Oil is used around the world for a variety of uses; acne, skin lesions, burns, fungal infections (e.g., of the toenail), herpes, eczema, leg sores, bed sores, gingivitis, hemorrhoids, STD's, cold sores, and many others.

This appears to be the only way to stabilize ozone without adding artificial stabilizers, chemicals or preservatives. Ozone is bubbled at very high concentrations, under a controlled environment for days until it slowly begins to solidify. This solid form of olive oil forms a Vaseline or salve like substance and will keep for many months on the shelf. If kept refrigerated, it maintains its full effectiveness almost indefinitely. Some individuals even choose to ingest ozonated olive oil in order to obtain the system-wide effects of using ozone medically.

Bagging

"Bagging" with ozone refers to the method of isolating a body part by surrounding it with a bag (such as hand, arm, leg, foot, torso, pelvis, but never the head), and introducing ozone. This can be used to treat gangrene, diabetic foot ulcers, bed sores, burns, any wounds that are infected or slow healing, or those that refuse to heal. This method is not intended to generate an immune modulating effect on the individual as in the methods above.

The bag is placed around or over the affected area, and the output tube from the ozone generator placed through the top of the bag, and the top sealed as effectively as possible. Ozone at the desired concentration must first be humidified, (simply bubble through the water) and then it enters the bag, as the ozone generator constantly runs during this treatment.

Treatment times vary depending on the type of wounds being treated but typically range from ten-thirty minutes. As leaking will occur from the bag, it is suggested that this process occur in a well-ventilated area. After the treatment the bag will still contain a high concentration of ozone, which is irritating to the lungs, nose, and eyes if it escapes from the bag. This is usually disposed of in a safe manner. In European Medical Clinics, a specially designed bag is used to ensure no leaking occurs, and after treatment the ozone is sucked from the bag by a vacuum pump so neither the patient nor the attendant ever breathes in the ozone.

In this method the ozone kills any bacteria, viruses, fungus or molds infecting the open wound, increase blood flow to the wound and stimulating the healing process. It has been documented that many a body part has been spared amputation through the application of ozone in this method.

High concentrations of ozone applied through bagging (60-90ug/ml) tend to have a sterilization effect on the wound, but if used for prolonged periods will have a negative effect on healing. Mild-range ozone concentrations (30-40ug/ ml) will have a healing effect on the wounds. Therefore the protocol as suggested by German researchers is to begin with the infected wound at 75-90ug/ml for the sterilizing effect, and as the treatments begin to clear the wound of infection, to gradually drop the concentration towards 35ug/ml. This gradual drop in the concentration will maintain the sterility of the wound and stimulate healing. Individual differences in this protocol are taken into account by watching the effect of the ozone on the wound, and the rate at which it closes.

Major autohemotherapy

This procedure is performed only by trained professionals, usually in a clinic setting. Approximately 200cc of the patient's blood is withdrawn into an evacuated bottle. The bottle is then hung upside down, and ozone gas (the same volume as the blood withdrawn) is infused into the bottle, usually at a concentration of 40ug/ml. The blood is then given back to the patient, much like a transfusion.

In this procedure the trained professional constantly monitors' the patient, and ensures the purity of the ozone gas, and the sterility of all equipment used. For the trained professional this treatment is actually quite easy, and very safe for the patient.

Major autohemotherapy is the preferred method of many practitioners, and it is used in well over 150 diseases. In Germany, even the ambulances are equipped with ozone generators. If ozone is administered within twenty-four hours of a stroke, 95% of patients suffer no permanent paralysis.

Enhancing the outcome of ozone therapy

- Nutritional supplements
- Therapeutic nutrition
- Chelation therapy
- Chiropractic support

The author deals with this subject more extensively in a 300-page book, The Impact of Ozone on Health, soon to be published in Malaysia. He maintains that whereas ozone can achieve results as shown in this book, the results can be dramatically maximized when ozone is supported with lifestyle changes, therapeutic nutrition, detoxification, posture and breathing. He emphasizes that these results need to be sustained following the initial success. Patients who are treated with ozone are already suffering from malnutrition (from poor diet or inadequate nutrition), weak immune system and mental/ emotional stress. He cites experience where the treatment of degenerative diseases including cancer, as well as AIDs patients, recover more quickly and sustain recovery as compared to those treated with ozone only. He maintains that the potential to heal as well as achieve extended youthful aging, is becoming a science directing the patient to apply a lifestyle change, nutrition, posture and breathing, as well as a new approach to confronting emotional stress.

Application of research studies relating to nutritional deficiencies leads to more predictable results when using these protocols; antioxidants and the enhancing effect of vitamins E, A, C and selenium, a B complex, zinc, as well as a other specific supplements such as N-acetyl-cysteine, depending on individual circumstances. Therapeutic nutrition — meaning an individually packaged program developed for each patient determined by tests revealing nutritional deficiencies — is an effective way to address disease conditions.

The Use Of Chelation Therapy In Combination with Ozone

Medical doctors are reporting additional benefits when chelating is combined with ozone. The chelating administered intravenously includes vitamin B complex, vitamin C and trace minerals. Whereas chelation is used to treat heart disease for many years, reports of the use of chelating to treat a number of other diseases continues to be increasingly more impressive.

A study conducted at the Ozone Research Centre reports the following: Patients with cardiac infarction show a decrease in glutathione peroxidase and superoxide dismutase activities, which are precursors in the scavenger processes of lipid peroxide and superoxide radicals, respectively. This study investigated the effects of endovenous ozone therapy on serum lipid pattern and on antioxidant defense system, such as the glutathione redox, in the blood of patients with myocardial infarct. Twenty-two patients who had an infarction, between three months and one year before the study, were treated with ozone by autohemotherapy during fifteen sessions. A statistically significant decrease in plasma total cholesterol and low density lipoprotein was observed. High peroxidase and glucose 6-phosphate dehydrogenase activities were found. There was no change in plasma lipid peroxidation levels. It was concluded that endovenous ozone therapy in patients with myocardial infarction activates the antioxidant protection system.

An example of the extent of ozone application is reported in a breakthrough treatment of herniated disks described as the Discosan Method. In Italy, orthopedic surgeons who used to perform surgery on herniated discs are now using a special mixture of ozone to treat the pathology of this condition. Developed by Dr. Cesare Verga (orthopedic surgeon) who developed the system in 1984 has treated over 6,000 patients. Dr. Verga claims that surgery really does not address the underlying cause. As a matter of fact it offsets the biomechanics of the spine. Ozone as administered in the Discosan Method, represents a new approach in the treatment of herniated discs which resolves the biological and biomedical aspect of the pathology. Dr. Verga states that this approach has a success rate of over 95%. Some of the principal characteristics that make this method so unique are the following:

- No contra indications
- Over 95% success rates
- Virtually zero recovery time with no side effects

The treatment consists of injections of a special mixture of ozone and oxygen administered around the herniated zone. The success of this application has been successful even when surgery had not corrected the problem.

The Potential of Ozone in Your Clinic

The information below provides a summary of selected information for those interested in ozone and integrated health care. Medical doctors interested in introducing ozone are invited to apply for a Questionnaire. In response you will receive an invitation to see a demonstration of the ozone therapy being administered at an approved center.

Acariasis	Acne	Acrodermatitis
Acuteotitis media	Acute vestibulopathy	Addisons disease
Adenocarcinoma	Adenovirus	Adrenalitis
AIDS	Allergies	Alopecia
ALS (Low Gehrig disease)	Alzheimer's disease	Amebiasis
Amenorrhoea	Amyloidosis	Anal Fissures
Anemia	Angina	Angiodema
Ankylosing Spondylitis	Anthrax	Apthous Stomatitis
Arterial occlusion	Arteriosclerosis	Arthritis

Arthrosis	Asthma	Athlete's foot
Babesiosis	Bacterial Pneumonia	Bartonellosis
Bell's Palsy	Bornholm myalgia	Botulism
Bronchitis	Bronchopulmonary aspergilus	Bronchospasm
Brucellosis	Bullous pemphigus	Burkit lymphoma
All types of cancer	Candidiasis	Carbuncles
Cavernous sinus thrombosis	Cellulitis	Cerebral atrophy
Cerebro vascular accident injuries	Chagas disease	Chicken pox
Chlamydia	Cholecystitis	Chronic pain
Chronic pulmonary disease	Cirrhosis of the liver	Coccidiomycosis
Colitis	Colorado tick fever	Conjunctivitis
Contact dermatitis	Coronavirus	Cryoglobulinemia
Cryptococcosis	Cryptospiridiosis	Cutaneous larva migrans
Cystitis	Cytomegalovirus	Dengue fever
Dermatitis	Diabetes	Diverticulits
Echovirus	Eczema	Ehrlichiosis
Emphysema	Encephalitis	Encephalomyelitis
Endocarditis	Endometritis	Endophthalmitis
Enteric fever	Enteritis necroticans	Environmental sensitivity
Epidermoid carcinoma	Epidermolytic keratosis	Epidermophytosis
Epididymitis	Epstein-Barr virus	Erysipelas
Erythema migrans	Flativirus	Folliculitis
Food poisoning	Fulminant varicella	Furuncle
Gangrene	Genital warts	Giardiasis
Glaucoma	Glioma	Glomerular membrane disease

Glommerulo-nephritis	Goodpasture syndrome	Gout
Graves Disease	Guillan-Barre syndrome	Haemotoma
Haemorrhage	Haemorrhagic fever	Hairy leukplakia
Heart arrhythmia	Heart disease	Hemorrhoids
Hepatitis	All types of Herpes	Histoplasmosis
HIV	HTLV	Huntingdon chorea
Hypercholosterolem	Hypersensitivity	Hyperthyroidism
Hypotension	Ichthyosis	Ileitis
Impetigo	Influenza	Intravascular coagulation
Ischemic optic neuropathy	Krohn's disease	Kyanasur Forest disease
Landry syndrome	Lassa fever	Leishmaniasis
Leptospirosis	Leukopenia	Leukemia
Leukoence-phalopathy	Listeriosis	Liver disfunction
Lupus erythemalosus	Lyme disease	Lymphocytic choriomeningitis
Lympho-granuloma	Lymphoid pneumonia	Lymphoma
Malaria	Mastoiditis	Measles
Melanoma	Melioidosis	Meniere's disease
Migraine	Moluscum ecthyma	Mononucleosis
Morbilloform	Multiple sclerosis	Mumps
Myalgia	Myasthenia gravis	Mycobacterium avium complex
Mycosis	Myeltis	Mycarditis
Myonecrosis	Myositis	Neurodermatitis
Neutropenia colitis	Ocular trachoma	Optic nerve dysfunction
Optic neuritis	Oral erythema	Orbital cellulitis
Orchitis	Osteomyelitis	Osteoporosis

Osteosarcoma	Otosclerosis	Pancreatitis
Panniculitis	Papillitis	Parainfluenza
Parkinson's disease	Pediculosis	Pelvic inflammatory disease
Pemphigoid	Pernicious anemia	Pneumocytosis
Pneumonia	Poliomyelitis	Polyateritis
Polyoma virus	Poor circulation	Postpartum fever
Proctitis	Prostate enlargement	Prurigo
Psoriasis	Pulmonary toxiplasis	Pyoderma
Rabies	Radioculoneuritis	Relapsing fever
Reynaud's disease	Reynold's syndrome	Rheumatism
Rheumatoid arthritis	Rhinitis	Rift Valley fever
Rubella	Salmonella	Salpingitis
Scabies	Scleroderma	Senile dementia
Senile macular degeneration	Sennutsu fever	Septicaemia
Shingles	Shock	Sickle cell anemia
Sinusitis	Skin burns	Spinalioma
Staphyloccus	Stomatiis	Striatonigral degeneration
Stroke	Syphillis	T. cruzi
Tardive dyskinesia	Tendinitis	Tetanus
Thoracic zygomycosis	Thrombopenic purpura	Thrombophlebitis
Thryroiditis	Tinea versicolor	Tinnitis
Togavirus	Tourette syndrome	Toxic amblyopia
Toxoplasmosis	Traveller's diarrhea	Trench fever
Trypanosomiasis	Tuberculosis	Tularaemia
Ulcers	Urethritis	Urticaria

Uterine spasm	Uveitis	Varicella pneumonia
Varicose veins	Vasculitis	Vascular retinopathy
Warts	Wegener granulomatosis	

References

R. Radel and M.H. Navidi, Chemistry (81. Paul: West Publishing, 1990).

S.S. Hendler, The Oxygen Breakthrough (New York: Pocket Books, 1989).

M. Barry and M. Cullen, "The Air You Breathe Up There." Conde Nast Traveller, December 1993.

Otto Warburg. The Prime Cause and Prevention of Cancer (Wurzburg K. Triltsch, 1 966).

Encyclopedia, 7th edition volume 2 (New York; Van Nostrand Reinhold, 1989).

Natalie Angier, "The Price We Pay for Breathing." The New York Times Magazine, April 25, 1993).

David Lin, Free Radicals and Disease Prevention (New Canaan, Conn. Keats Publishing, 1993).

Sara Shannon, Good Health in a Toxic World: The Complete Guide to Fighting Free Radicals (New York: Warner Books, 1994).

Stephen A. Levine and Parris M. Kidd, Antioxidant Adaption (San Leandro, California: Allergy Research Corporation, 1986).

Marie Theres Jacobs, "Adverse Effects and typical Complications in OzoneOxygen Therapy," Ozonachrichten (1982).

"The Intravenous Use of Hydrogen Peroxide," The Lancet, February 21, 1920.

Oxidative Therapy (Oklahoma City: International Bio- Oxidative Medicine Foundation, n.d.).

Frank Shallenberger, "Intravenous Ozone Therapy in HIV Relted Disease," Proceedings: Fourth International Bio- Oxidative Medical Conference, April 1993.

M.T. Carpendale, interview in Ozone and the Politics of Medicine (Vancouver; Threshold Film1993).

Horst Kief, interview in Ozone and the Politics of Medicine

(Vancouver; Threshold Film, 1993):

The Value Line Investment Survey 69, no. 8 (November 5, 1993).

Chemical Technology: An Encyclopedic Treatment, vol. 1 (New York: Barnes and Noble, 1968).

Siegfried Rilling and Renate Viebahn, The Use of Ozone in Medicine (Heidelberg: Haug Publishers, 1987).

A.C. Baggs, "Are Worry-Free Transfusions just a Whiff of Ozone Away?" Canadian Medical Association Journal (April 1, 1993).

"Family Medicine Nation," Journal of Public Health Policy, 12, no. 1 (Spring 1991).

Andres Oppenheimer, Castro's Final Hour (New York; Touchstone Books, 1993).

McGraw-Hili Encyclopedia of Science and Technology, 3rd ed., vol, 16, (New York: McGraw-Hill, 1987).

Othmer, Encyclopedia of Chemical Technology, 3rd ed., vol. 16 (New York: John Wiley and Sons, 1981).

Proceedings of the First Ibero/Latinamerican Congress Research, 1990).

Revista CENIC Ciencias Biol6gicas, 20, no 1-2-3 (1989).

Silvia Menendez, Ozomed/Ozone Therapy (Havana:)

Fritz Kramer, "Ozone in the Dental Practice," in Medical Applications of Ozone, edited by Julius LaRaus (Norwalk, Conn: Internation~1 Ozone Association, Pan American Committee, 1983).

Gerad Sunnen, "Ozone in Medicine: Overview and Future Direction," Journal of Advancementin Medicine 1, no. 3 (Fall 1988).

S.N. Gorbunov et al. "The Use of Ozone in the Treatment of Children Suffered Due to Different Catastrophies" in Ozone in Medicine: Proceedings Eleventh Ozone World Congress (Stamford, Conn: International Ozone Association, Pan American Committee, 1993).

Horst Kief, The Autohomologous Immune Therapy, monograph, (Ludwigshafen: Kief Clinic, 1992).

Ed McCabe, Oxygen Therapies (Morrisville, N. Y. Energy Publications, 1988).

Anthony di Fabio, Supplement to the Art of Getting Well (Franklin, Tenn. The Rheumatoid Disease Foundation, 1989).

C. H. Farr, Protocol for the Intravenous Administration of Hydrogen Peroxide (Oklahoma City: International Bio- Oxidative MediCine Foundation, 1993).

J. Varro, "Ozone Applications in Cancer Cases," Medical Applications of Ozone, (Norwalk, Conn.: International Ozone Association, Pan American Committee, 1983.

Paul. Sergios, One Boy at War: My Life in the AIDS Underground (New York, Alfred A. Knopf, 1993).

F. Sweet et al., "Ozone Selectively Inhibits Growth of Cancer Cells," Science 209 (August 22, 1980).

Betsy Russell-Manning, ed., Self-treatment for Aids, Oxygen Therapies, etc. (San Francisco: Greenwood Press; 1988).

B.L. Aronoff et al., Regional Oxygenation in Neoplasms," Cancer, 18 (October 1965).

M. Arnan, and L.E. DeVries, "Effect of Ozone/Oxygen Gas Mixture Directly Injected into the Mammary Carcinoma of the Female C3H/HEJ Mice," in Medical Applications oDengue feverf Ozone, edited by Julius LaRaus (Norwalk, Conn. International Ozone Association Pan American Committee, 1983).

L. Paulesu et al., "Studies on the Biological Effects of Ozone: 2 Induction of Tumor Necrosis Factor on Human Leucocytes," Lymphakine and Cytakine Research 10 no. 5 (1991).

M. T. Carpendale and J. K. Freeberg, "Ozone Inactivates HIV at Non-Cytotoxic Concentrations," Antiviral Research 16 (1991).

About the Author

Dr. Jacob Swilling is a noted research scientist, author of several books, and the founder of several natural alternative health clinics in the U.S. and other countries, including Malaysia, Mexico, and South Africa. His mission is to share twenty-five years of research experience working with thousands of patients seeking self-help through applying natural healing methods to maximize the successful outcome of the medical experience.

Dr. Swilling currently operates Know Your Options Wellness Resource Center, in Costa Mesa, California. He also serves as a consultant to physicians and healthcare practitioners, and a network of Know Your Options coordinators throughout the U.S., providing information, training, health assessments, and health monitoring, as well as other support services. He is also consultant to the Bio-Medical Cancer Center in Baja, Mexico, and coordinates a Cancer Self-Help Support program for patients returning to the U.S.

Other books by Dr. Swilling:

pH, HCL and Blood Sugar as Determining Factors in Health and Disease

Diabetes: A Self-Help Solution

Minerals: Key to Vibrant Health and Life Force

Healing Power of Natural Whole Foods

Cancer Self-Help Support Program

Nutrition, Sex and Fertility

Guidelines for Planning a Nutritious and Balanced Daily Diet

Bio-Cleanse Detoxification and Colon Restoration Program

Self-Help Breakthrough to Help the Body Heal Itself

For further information contact KYO Publishing at 714-708-3600

29761400R00027

Made in the USA
Middletown, DE
02 March 2016